CLINICAL LABORATORY MEDICINE PEARLS

A Comprehensive Guide

Dr Essam Abdelhakim

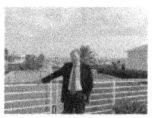

Copyright © 2024 Dr Essam Abdelhakim

All rights reserved

The characters and events portrayed in this book are fictitious. Any similarity to real persons, living or dead, is coincidental and not intended by the author.

No part of this book may be reproduced, or stored in a retrieval system, or transmitted in any form or by any means, electronic, mechanical, photocopying, recording, or otherwise, without express written permission of the publisher.

Cover design by: Art Painter
Library of Congress Control Number: 2018675309
Printed in the United States of America

CONTENTS

Title Page
Copyright
Disclosure
Introduction   1
Normal Reference Ranges and Factors Influencing Variability 2
Chapter 2: Full Blood Count (FBC)   7
Chapter 3: Renal Profile   14
Chapter 4: Liver Profile   23
Chapter 5: Bone Profile   31
Chapter 6: Lipid Profile   39
Chapter 7: Thyroid Function Tests   46
Chapter 8: Inflammatory Markers   54
Chapter 9: Coagulation Profiles   63
Chapter 10: Advanced Biochemical Tests   71
Chapter 11: Integrating Laboratory Results with Clinical Context   78
About The Author   85

DISCLOSURE

Disclosure

This book has been created with the assistance of *Artificial Intelligence (AI) tools* and thoroughly reviewed and edited by the author to ensure clarity, relevance, and educational value.

While every effort has been made to provide accurate and up-to-date information, this content is intended solely for educational and informational purposes.

The author is a medical professional; however, the information provided in this book *is not a substitute for professional medical advice, diagnosis, or treatment.*

Readers are strongly advised to consult licensed healthcare providers or specialists for any medical concerns or conditions.

By using this book, **you acknowledge and agree** that the author shall not be held responsible or liable for any loss, damage, or harm whether physical, emotional, financial, or otherwise that may occur *as a result of the use or misuse of the information presented herein.*

INTRODUCTION

In this book, we aim to provide a comprehensive and practical guide to understanding and interpreting key laboratory investigations.

The focus is on commonly used tests such as **full blood count (FBC), renal profile, liver profile, and bone profile**, among others.

Each section delves into the individual components of these tests, explores their clinical significance, and outlines the potential causes of abnormal results.

By linking these abnormalities to differential diagnoses, the book equips clinicians with the knowledge needed to approach complex clinical scenarios systematically.

Who Is This Book For?

- **Primary care physicians and general practitioners** who need to interpret a wide range of tests in outpatient settings.
- **Specialists** who rely on specific profiles, such as nephrologists for renal tests or hepatologists for liver assessments.
- **Medical students and trainees** seeking to build a strong foundation in laboratory medicine.
- **Allied healthcare professionals** involved in patient care, such as nurse practitioners, physician assistants, and clinical pharmacists.

NORMAL REFERENCE RANGES AND FACTORS INFLUENCING VARIABILITY

1. **Normal Reference Ranges**
   - **Definition:** The normal reference range is typically derived from testing a healthy population and includes the central 95% of values.
     - Example: Normal hemoglobin for adult males is approximately 13.5–17.5 g/dL, while for females, it is 12.0–15.5 g/dL.
   - **Limitations:**
     - Reference ranges may not apply universally across populations or clinical scenarios.
     - Extremes of the range (e.g., the upper 2.5% or lower 2.5%) may still represent normal physiology for certain individuals.

2. **Factors Influencing Variability**

Several factors affect laboratory test results, and clinicians must consider these when interpreting values:

- **Age:**
  - Neonates often have higher bilirubin levels due to immature liver function.
  - Older adults may show altered renal function with reduced eGFR, even in the absence of overt kidney disease.
- **Sex:**
  - Hormonal differences influence lab values. For instance, males generally have higher

hemoglobin levels than females due to androgen-stimulated erythropoiesis.
- **Race and Ethnicity:**
    - African Americans may have lower baseline white blood cell (WBC) counts compared to other populations.
    - Differences in creatinine kinase (CK) levels are observed across ethnicities due to muscle mass variability.
- **Physiological Status:**
    - Fasting vs. non-fasting can significantly impact glucose and lipid profile results.
    - Stress, dehydration, or recent physical activity can transiently alter lab values.
- **Medications:**
    - Certain drugs can directly affect lab values, either by altering the analyte or by interfering with the assay. For example:
        - Diuretics can cause hypokalemia.
        - Proton pump inhibitors (PPIs) can lead to hypomagnesemia.
- **Methodological Factors:**
    - Different laboratories use varying techniques and equipment, leading to slight variations in reference ranges.

3. Clinical Context Is Key

- Lab results must always be interpreted in conjunction with the clinical context, patient history, and physical examination findings.
- For example, a low TSH level may indicate hyperthyroidism in an outpatient setting but could also be a transient finding during acute illness (non-

thyroidal illness syndrome).

Principles Of Differential Diagnosis Using Lab Results

The following principles guide the process:

1. Understand the Pathophysiology
- Each lab result reflects a physiological or pathological process. For example:
  - Elevated alkaline phosphatase may indicate increased bone turnover (e.g., Paget's disease) or cholestasis (e.g., biliary obstruction).

2. Determine the Pattern of Abnormalities
- Isolated vs. grouped abnormalities can provide clues:
  - Isolated thrombocytopenia suggests immune thrombocytopenic purpura (ITP).
  - Combined anemia, leukopenia, and thrombocytopenia may indicate bone marrow failure.

3. Consider Clinical Correlation
- Correlate lab abnormalities with symptoms and physical findings. For instance:
  - Elevated creatinine with oliguria suggests acute kidney injury.
  - High bilirubin with jaundice and dark urine points to liver dysfunction or hemolysis.

4. Generate a Differential Diagnosis
- Categorize causes into broad groups:
  - **Physiological vs. pathological:** E.g., transient neutrophilia due to stress vs. neutrophilia from bacterial infection.
  - **Primary vs. secondary:** Hyperparathyroidism due to parathyroid

adenoma (primary) vs. chronic kidney disease (secondary).
- **Acute vs. chronic:** Elevated transaminases from acute hepatitis vs. cirrhosis.

5. Use a Stepwise Diagnostic Approach
- Begin with the most common and treatable conditions, ruling out life-threatening causes early.
  - For hypercalcemia: Start with primary hyperparathyroidism, then consider malignancy, granulomatous diseases, or drug effects.

6. Recognize Artifacts and Pitfalls
- Be aware of pre-analytical, analytical, and post-analytical errors:
  - Hemolysis during sample collection can falsely elevate potassium levels.
  - Lipemia may interfere with the measurement of certain analytes like glucose or triglycerides.

7. Follow-Up and Monitor Trends
- Repeating tests or monitoring changes over time can clarify ambiguous findings. For example:
  - Persistent mild transaminase elevation may warrant additional testing for viral hepatitis or autoimmune liver disease.

CHAPTER 2: FULL BLOOD COUNT (FBC)

Components Of The Fbc

1. Hemoglobin (Hb):
- Measures the oxygen-carrying capacity of red blood cells.
- Normal ranges:
    - Adult males: 13.5–17.5 g/dL
    - Adult females: 12.0–15.5 g/dL
    - Children: 11.0–16.0 g/dL

2. Hematocrit (Hct):
- Represents the percentage of blood volume occupied by RBCs.
- Normal ranges:
    - Adult males: 41–53%
    - Adult females: 36–46%
    - Children: 35–45%

3. Red Blood Cell Count (RBC):
- Reflects the total number of RBCs in a given volume of blood.
- Normal ranges:
    - Adult males: 4.7–6.1 million/µL
    - Adult females: 4.2–5.4 million/µL
    - Children: 4.1–5.5 million/µL

4. Red Cell Indices:
- **Mean Corpuscular Volume (MCV):** Average size of RBCs (normal: 80–100 fL).
  - Microcytic: MCV < 80 fL.
  - Macrocytic: MCV > 100 fL.
- **Mean Corpuscular Hemoglobin (MCH):** Average Hb per RBC (normal: 27–31 pg).
- **Mean Corpuscular Hemoglobin Concentration (MCHC):** Average Hb concentration in RBCs (normal: 32–36 g/dL).
- **Red Cell Distribution Width (RDW):** Measure of variability in RBC size. Elevated in conditions like iron deficiency anemia and mixed anemia.

5. White Blood Cell Count (WBC):
- Reflects the total number of leukocytes.
- Normal range: 4,000–11,000/μL.

6. Platelet Count:
- Indicates the number of platelets, which are essential for coagulation.
- Normal range: 150,000–450,000/μL.

Causes Of Abnormalities In Fbc

1. Anemia
Anemia refers to a reduction in hemoglobin concentration, RBC count, or hematocrit, leading to decreased oxygen delivery to tissues.

Based on MCV, anemia is classified as:

A. Microcytic Anemia (Mcv < 80 Fl)

Common Causes:

- **Iron deficiency anemia:** Most common cause; associated with chronic blood loss, poor dietary intake, or malabsorption.
- **Thalassemias:** Genetic disorders causing reduced or absent synthesis of globin chains.
- **Anemia of chronic disease:** Chronic inflammation reduces iron availability.
- **Lead poisoning:** Disrupts heme synthesis.
- **Sideroblastic anemia:** Impaired incorporation of iron into heme.

B. Macrocytic Anemia (Mcv > 100 Fl)

Common Causes:

- **Vitamin B12 deficiency:** Often due to pernicious anemia, malabsorption, or dietary deficiency.
- **Folate deficiency:** Seen in malnutrition, alcoholism, and pregnancy.
- **Liver disease:** Alters lipid composition of RBC membranes.
- **Hypothyroidism:** Reduces hematopoiesis.
- **Myelodysplastic syndromes:** Bone marrow dysfunction.

C. Normocytic Anemia (Mcv 80–100 Fl)

Common Causes:

- **Acute blood loss:** Reduces total RBC count.
- **Hemolytic anemia:** Increased destruction of RBCs (e.g., autoimmune hemolysis, sickle cell disease).
- **Anemia of chronic disease:** Inflammation suppresses

erythropoiesis.
- **Aplastic anemia:** Bone marrow failure due to radiation, toxins, or autoimmune causes.

2. White Blood Cell Abnormalities

A. Leukocytosis (Wbc > 11,000/Ml)

Common Causes:
- **Infections:** Bacterial infections often cause neutrophilia, while viral infections may cause lymphocytosis.
- **Leukemias:** Elevated blasts in acute leukemia or mature cells in chronic leukemias.
- **Inflammation:** Rheumatoid arthritis, vasculitis.
- **Stress response:** Physical or emotional stress elevates WBC count.
- **Medications:** Corticosteroids can cause neutrophilia.

B. Leukopenia (Wbc < 4,000/Ml)

Common Causes:
- **Viral infections:** Suppress bone marrow temporarily.
- **Bone marrow disorders:** Aplastic anemia, leukemia, or myelodysplastic syndromes.
- **Drugs:** Chemotherapy, immunosuppressants, and certain antibiotics.
- **Autoimmune diseases:** Lupus, Felty's syndrome.
- **Nutritional deficiencies:** Vitamin B12 or folate deficiency.

3. Platelet Abnormalities

A. Thrombocytopenia (Platelets < 150,000/Ml)

Common Causes:

- **Bone marrow failure:** Aplastic anemia, myelodysplastic syndromes.
- **Infections:** Dengue, HIV, or sepsis.
- **Autoimmune diseases:** Immune thrombocytopenic purpura (ITP), systemic lupus erythematosus.
- **Splenic sequestration:** Portal hypertension, splenomegaly.
- **Medications:** Heparin-induced thrombocytopenia (HIT).

B. Thrombocytosis (Platelets > 450,000/Ml)

Common Causes:

- **Reactive thrombocytosis:** Infections, inflammation, or iron deficiency.
- **Myeloproliferative disorders:** Essential thrombocythemia, polycythemia vera.
- **Post-splenectomy:** Transient thrombocytosis following splenic removal.

Differential Diagnosis And Case-Based Discussions

Case 1: Microcytic Anemia In A 35-Year-Old Female

- **Presentation:** Fatigue, pallor, and heavy menstrual periods.
- **FBC Findings:** Hb 9 g/dL, MCV 70 fL, RDW elevated.
- **Diagnosis:** Iron deficiency anemia due to chronic blood loss.
- **Key Takeaway:** Always investigate underlying causes of anemia.

Case 2: Leukocytosis In A 60-Year-Old Male With Fever

- **Presentation:** Fever, cough, and shortness of breath.
- **FBC Findings:** WBC 18,000/μL with neutrophilia.
- **Diagnosis:** Bacterial pneumonia.
- **Key Takeaway:** WBC differential is critical in identifying infection type.

Case 3: Thrombocytopenia In A 50-Year-Old Male On Heparin

- **Presentation:** Post-operative patient develops bruising and low platelet count.
- **FBC Findings:** Platelets 90,000/μL.
- **Diagnosis:** Heparin-induced thrombocytopenia (HIT).
- **Key Takeaway:** Monitor platelet counts closely in patients receiving heparin.

Case 4: Pancytopenia In A 45-Year-Old Female

- **Presentation:** Fatigue, bruising, and recurrent infections.
- **FBC Findings:** Low Hb, WBC, and platelets.
- **Diagnosis:** Aplastic anemia.
- **Key Takeaway:** Bone marrow evaluation is essential in pancytopenia.

CHAPTER 3: RENAL PROFILE

Key Markers In The Renal Profile

1. Urea
- **Source:** Produced in the liver as a byproduct of protein metabolism.
- **Normal Range:** 2.5–7.1 mmol/L (7–20 mg/dL).
- **Clinical Significance:**
    - **Increased Urea (Azotemia):**
        - **Prerenal:** Dehydration, hypovolemia, heart failure.
        - **Renal:** Acute kidney injury (AKI), chronic kidney disease (CKD).
        - **Postrenal:** Obstruction (e.g., stones, prostate hypertrophy).
    - **Decreased Urea:** Severe liver disease, malnutrition, or low protein intake.

2. Creatinine
- **Source:** A product of muscle metabolism excreted by the kidneys.
- **Normal Range:**
    - Adult males: 62–106 µmol/L (0.7–1.2 mg/dL).
    - Adult females: 44–80 µmol/L (0.5–1.0 mg/dL).
- **Clinical Significance:**
    - Elevated creatinine suggests impaired glomerular filtration.

- Less sensitive to early kidney dysfunction due to variations in muscle mass.

3. Estimated Glomerular Filtration Rate (Egfr)

- **Purpose:** Provides an estimate of kidney filtration efficiency.
- **Calculation:** Based on serum creatinine, age, sex, and race.
- **Normal Range:** ≥90 mL/min/1.73 m².
- **Clinical Significance:**
    - **Mild CKD:** eGFR 60–89 mL/min.
    - **Moderate CKD:** eGFR 30–59 mL/min.
    - **Severe CKD:** eGFR <30 mL/min.
    - **End-Stage Renal Disease (ESRD):** eGFR <15 mL/min.

4. Electrolytes

- **Sodium (Na⁺):** Normal range: 135–145 mmol/L.
    - Key roles: Fluid balance, nerve impulse conduction.
    - Imbalances: Hyponatremia, hypernatremia.
- **Potassium (K⁺):** Normal range: 3.5–5.0 mmol/L.
    - Key roles: Muscle contraction, cardiac function.
    - Imbalances: Hyperkalemia, hypokalemia.
- **Chloride (Cl⁻):** Normal range: 98–106 mmol/L.
    - Maintains acid-base balance.

- **Bicarbonate (HCO_3^-):** Normal range: 22–28 mmol/L.
  ◦ Indicates acid-base status.

Clinical Interpretation Of Renal Profile

1. Acute Kidney Injury (Aki) Vs. Chronic Kidney Disease (Ckd)

- **Acute Kidney Injury (AKI):**
    - Rapid decline in kidney function.
    - Hallmark: Rising creatinine and decreased urine output.
    - **Causes:**
        - **Prerenal:** Hypovolemia, hypotension.
        - **Renal:** Acute tubular necrosis (ATN), glomerulonephritis.
        - **Postrenal:** Urinary tract obstruction.
    - **Key Markers:** Elevated creatinine, hyperkalemia, acidosis.
- **Chronic Kidney Disease (CKD):**
    - Gradual loss of kidney function over months/years.
    - Hallmark: Persistent eGFR <60 mL/min for >3 months.
    - **Causes:** Diabetes, hypertension, chronic glomerulonephritis, polycystic kidney disease.
    - **Key Markers:** Elevated creatinine and urea, electrolyte imbalances, anemia, secondary hyperparathyroidism.

2. Electrolyte Imbalances

A. Hyperkalemia (K⁺ > 5.0 Mmol/L)

- **Causes:**
    - **Reduced Excretion:** AKI, CKD, adrenal insufficiency.
    - **Shift from Cells to Plasma:** Acidosis, hemolysis, rhabdomyolysis.
    - **Medications:** ACE inhibitors, ARBs, potassium-sparing diuretics.
- **Clinical Manifestations:** Muscle weakness, cardiac arrhythmias (e.g., peaked T waves on ECG).

B. Hypokalemia (K⁺ < 3.5 Mmol/L)

- **Causes:**
    - **Increased Loss:** Diuretics, vomiting, diarrhea.
    - **Intracellular Shift:** Alkalosis, insulin administration.
- **Clinical Manifestations:** Muscle cramps, weakness, arrhythmias (e.g., U waves on ECG).

C. Hyponatremia (Na⁺ < 135 Mmol/L)

- **Causes:**
    - **Hypovolemic:** Vomiting, diarrhea, diuretics.
    - **Euvolemic:** SIADH, hypothyroidism.
    - **Hypervolemic:** Heart failure, cirrhosis, nephrotic syndrome.
- **Clinical Manifestations:** Confusion, seizures, coma.

D. Hypernatremia (Na⁺ > 145 Mmol/L)

- **Causes:**
  - **Water Loss:** Diabetes insipidus, excessive sweating.
  - **Sodium Gain:** Hypertonic saline infusion.
- **Clinical Manifestations:** Lethargy, irritability, seizures.

3. Acid-Base Disturbances

A. Metabolic Acidosis

- **Causes:**
  - Increased acid production (e.g., ketoacidosis, lactic acidosis).
  - Loss of bicarbonate (e.g., diarrhea, renal tubular acidosis).
- **Key Marker:** Low bicarbonate (<22 mmol/L), low pH.

B. Metabolic Alkalosis

- **Causes:**
  - Loss of hydrogen ions (e.g., vomiting, diuretics).
  - Excess bicarbonate administration.
- **Key Marker:** Elevated bicarbonate (>28 mmol/L), high pH.

C. Respiratory Acidosis/Alkalosis

- Respiratory components (CO_2) indirectly reflected in bicarbonate levels.

Differential Diagnosis And Approach To Renal Dysfunction

Step 1: Evaluate Renal Function Parameters
- Check creatinine, urea, eGFR.
- Compare with baseline results to differentiate acute vs. chronic dysfunction.

Step 2: Assess Electrolytes and Acid-Base Status
- Identify imbalances in sodium, potassium, bicarbonate.

Step 3: Integrate Clinical History
- **Prerenal:** Look for signs of dehydration or low perfusion.
- **Renal:** Consider nephrotoxic drugs, systemic diseases.
- **Postrenal:** Rule out obstruction with imaging or clinical signs.

Step 4: Investigate Underlying Causes
- Use urinary studies (e.g., urinary sodium, creatinine clearance).
- Perform imaging (e.g., ultrasound, CT scan).
- Order specific tests (e.g., autoantibodies, complement levels) based on suspected diagnosis.

Case-Based Discussions

Case 1: Acute Kidney Injury In A Dehydrated Patient

- **Presentation:** Vomiting, decreased urine output.
- **Key Findings:** Elevated creatinine and urea, low eGFR.
- **Diagnosis:** Prerenal AKI due to dehydration.
- **Management:** Intravenous fluids to restore perfusion.

Case 2: Chronic Kidney Disease In A Diabetic Patient

- **Presentation:** Long-standing diabetes, fatigue, ankle swelling.
- **Key Findings:** eGFR 35 mL/min, normocytic anemia, hyperkalemia.
- **Diagnosis:** CKD secondary to diabetic nephropathy.
- **Management:** Glycemic control, ACE inhibitors, dietary modifications.

Case 3: Severe Hyperkalemia In A Patient On Ace Inhibitors

- **Presentation:** Muscle weakness, ECG showing peaked T waves.
- **Key Findings:** K^+ 6.5 mmol/L, normal creatinine.
- **Diagnosis:** Drug-induced hyperkalemia.
- **Management:** Discontinue ACE inhibitor, administer

calcium gluconate, and use potassium-lowering treatments.

CHAPTER 4: LIVER PROFILE

Markers Of Liver Function

1. Alanine Aminotransferase (ALT)

- **Source:** Primarily found in hepatocytes; released into the bloodstream when liver cells are damaged.
- **Normal Range:** 7–56 U/L.
- **Clinical Significance:**
  - **Elevated ALT:** Indicates hepatocellular injury, particularly in viral hepatitis, non-alcoholic fatty liver disease (NAFLD), or drug-induced liver injury.
  - More specific to the liver than AST.

2. Aspartate Aminotransferase (AST)

- **Source:** Found in the liver, cardiac muscle, and skeletal muscle.
- **Normal Range:** 10–40 U/L.
- **Clinical Significance:**
  - **Elevated AST:** Suggests liver injury but can also reflect damage to other tissues like the heart or muscles.
  - The **AST:ALT ratio** is clinically useful:
    - Ratio >2:1: Suggestive of alcoholic liver disease.
    - Ratio <1: Common in viral or non-alcoholic liver disease.

3. Alkaline Phosphatase (ALP)

- **Source:** Found in the liver, bile ducts, and bones.
- **Normal Range:** 44–147 U/L.
- **Clinical Significance:**
    - **Elevated ALP:** Associated with cholestasis, bile duct obstruction, or bone disorders.
    - A liver-specific cause can be confirmed if GGT is also elevated.

4. Gamma-Glutamyl Transferase (GGT)

- **Source:** Found in the liver and biliary tract.
- **Normal Range:** 0–51 U/L.
- **Clinical Significance:**
    - **Elevated GGT:** Suggests biliary or hepatic injury and is often used to confirm liver origin of elevated ALP.
    - Elevated in chronic alcohol use or certain medications (e.g., phenytoin).

5. Bilirubin

- **Source:** A breakdown product of hemoglobin metabolized by the liver and excreted in bile.
- **Normal Range:**
    - Total bilirubin: 0.3–1.2 mg/dL.
    - Direct bilirubin: 0–0.3 mg/dL.
- **Clinical Significance:**
    - **Unconjugated Hyperbilirubinemia:** Hemolysis, Gilbert's syndrome.
    - **Conjugated Hyperbilirubinemia:** Cholestasis, hepatocellular dysfunction, or

bile duct obstruction.

6. Albumin
- **Source:** Synthesized by the liver.
- **Normal Range:** 3.5–5.0 g/dL.
- **Clinical Significance:**
    - Low levels indicate reduced synthetic function in chronic liver disease, protein loss (e.g., nephrotic syndrome), or malnutrition.

7. Prothrombin Time (PT) / International Normalized Ratio (INR)
- **Source:** Reflects liver's ability to synthesize clotting factors.
- **Normal Range:**
    - PT: 10–13 seconds.
    - INR: 0.8–1.2.
- **Clinical Significance:**
    - Prolonged PT/INR suggests synthetic dysfunction, typically seen in advanced liver disease or vitamin K deficiency.

Patterns Of Liver Injury

1. Hepatocellular Pattern
- **Markers:** Elevated ALT and AST, often with ALT > AST (except in alcoholic liver disease).
- **Associated Conditions:**
    - Viral hepatitis (hepatitis A, B, C).
    - Non-alcoholic fatty liver disease (NAFLD).

- Drug-induced liver injury (e.g., paracetamol toxicity).

2. Cholestatic Pattern
- **Markers:** Elevated ALP and GGT, often with mild elevations in bilirubin.
- **Associated Conditions:**
    - Bile duct obstruction (e.g., gallstones, tumors).
    - Primary biliary cholangitis (PBC).
    - Primary sclerosing cholangitis (PSC).

3. Synthetic Dysfunction
- **Markers:** Low albumin, prolonged PT/INR.
- **Associated Conditions:**
    - Advanced cirrhosis.
    - Acute liver failure.
    - Vitamin K deficiency due to malabsorption.

Causes Of Abnormal Results

1. Viral Hepatitis
- **Pathophysiology:** Hepatic inflammation caused by viral infections (e.g., hepatitis A, B, C).
- **Key Findings:** Elevated ALT/AST (often ALT > AST), hyperbilirubinemia.
- **Differential Clue:**
    - Hepatitis A and E: Acute presentation.
    - Hepatitis B and C: Can progress to chronic liver disease or cirrhosis.

2. Alcoholic Liver Disease (ALD)

- **Pathophysiology:** Hepatic damage from chronic alcohol use.
- **Key Findings:** AST > ALT (typically >2:1), elevated GGT, macrocytic anemia.
- **Differential Clue:** History of alcohol abuse, presence of fatty liver or cirrhosis.

3. Non-Alcoholic Fatty Liver Disease (NAFLD)

- **Pathophysiology:** Fat accumulation in the liver associated with obesity, diabetes, or metabolic syndrome.
- **Key Findings:** Mildly elevated ALT > AST, normal or elevated ALP.
- **Differential Clue:** Absence of alcohol use, metabolic risk factors.

4. Cirrhosis

- **Pathophysiology:** Chronic scarring and liver dysfunction due to long-standing liver disease.
- **Key Findings:**
    - Low albumin.
    - Prolonged PT/INR.
    - Thrombocytopenia (due to splenic sequestration).
    - Elevated bilirubin in advanced disease.
- **Differential Clue:** Signs of portal hypertension (e.g., ascites, varices).

Differential Diagnosis And Interpretation Tips

Step 1: Analyze the Pattern of Liver Injury
- Hepatocellular: Look for ALT/AST elevations.
- Cholestatic: Check ALP and GGT levels.
- Synthetic dysfunction: Assess albumin and PT/INR.

Step 2: Correlate with Clinical History
- Consider patient's symptoms (e.g., jaundice, pruritus, abdominal pain).
- Review medications, alcohol use, and risk factors for viral hepatitis.

Step 3: Confirm the Diagnosis with Additional Tests
- Viral serologies (e.g., hepatitis B surface antigen, HCV RNA).
- Imaging (e.g., ultrasound, CT, or MRI) for structural abnormalities.
- Liver biopsy in uncertain or complex cases.

Case-Based Discussions

Case 1: Acute Viral Hepatitis

- **Presentation:** Fatigue, jaundice, right upper quadrant pain.
- **Key Findings:** ALT 800 U/L, AST 600 U/L, total bilirubin 3.2 mg/dL.
- **Diagnosis:** Hepatitis A.
- **Management:** Supportive care with monitoring of liver function.

Case 2: Alcoholic Liver Disease

- **Presentation:** Fatigue, abdominal swelling, history of alcohol use.
- **Key Findings:** AST 120 U/L, ALT 50 U/L, GGT 110 U/L, macrocytosis.
- **Diagnosis:** ALD with early cirrhosis.
- **Management:** Alcohol cessation, nutritional support, vitamin supplementation.

Case 3: Obstructive Jaundice Due To Gallstones

- **Presentation:** Jaundice, pale stools, dark urine, abdominal pain.
- **Key Findings:** ALP 400 U/L, GGT 200 U/L, conjugated bilirubin 4.5 mg/dL.

- **Diagnosis:** Choledocholithiasis.
- **Management:** Endoscopic retrograde cholangiopancreatography (ERCP) for stone removal.

CHAPTER 5: BONE PROFILE

Components Of The Bone Profile

1. Calcium (Total and Ionized)
- **Normal Ranges:**
    - Total calcium: 8.5–10.5 mg/dL.
    - Ionized calcium: 1.1–1.3 mmol/L (represents the biologically active fraction).
- **Clinical Significance:**
    - Total calcium is influenced by albumin levels; low albumin can cause pseudohypocalcemia.
    - Ionized calcium is unaffected by albumin and provides a more accurate measure of calcium status.
- **Functions:**
    - Essential for muscle contraction, nerve conduction, blood clotting, and bone health.

2. Phosphate
- **Normal Range:** 2.5–4.5 mg/dL.
- **Clinical Significance:**
    - Phosphate levels are regulated by the kidneys, PTH, and vitamin D.
    - High or low levels can indicate metabolic or renal disorders.

3. Alkaline Phosphatase (ALP)
- **Normal Range:** 44–147 U/L.

- **Clinical Significance:**
    - Produced by the liver and bones.
    - Elevated levels can indicate increased bone turnover, liver disease, or biliary obstruction.
    - In bone disease, the bone-specific ALP isoenzyme can help pinpoint the origin.

4. Vitamin D (25-Hydroxyvitamin D)
- **Normal Range:** 20–50 ng/mL.
- **Clinical Significance:**
    - Necessary for calcium absorption in the gut and bone mineralization.
    - Deficiency can lead to rickets in children or osteomalacia in adults.

5. Parathyroid Hormone (PTH)
- **Normal Range:** 10–65 pg/mL.
- **Clinical Significance:**
    - Regulates calcium and phosphate levels by acting on the bones, kidneys, and intestines.
    - Elevated PTH indicates primary or secondary hyperparathyroidism.

Electrolyte Disturbances

1. Hypercalcemia

Hypercalcemia is defined as serum calcium levels >10.5 mg/dL and is often associated with severe systemic effects if left untreated.

Causes:

- **Primary Hyperparathyroidism:**
    - Excess PTH production by the parathyroid glands.
    - Often due to a benign adenoma.
    - **Key Lab Findings:**
        - High calcium.
        - Low or normal phosphate.
        - Elevated PTH.
- **Malignancy-Associated Hypercalcemia:**
    - Caused by bone metastases or parathyroid hormone-related peptide (PTHrP) production by tumors.
    - Common in lung, breast, and renal cancers.
    - **Key Lab Findings:**
        - High calcium.
        - Low PTH.
        - Elevated PTHrP.
- **Granulomatous Diseases (e.g., Sarcoidosis, Tuberculosis):**
    - Increased conversion of vitamin D to its active form by macrophages.
    - **Key Lab Findings:**
        - High calcium.
        - Elevated vitamin D.

Clinical Features:

- Polyuria, polydipsia, constipation, fatigue, confusion, and, in severe cases, cardiac arrhythmias.

Management:

- Hydration with intravenous (IV) saline to promote renal calcium excretion.
- Bisphosphonates or denosumab to reduce bone resorption.
- Treat underlying cause (e.g., surgery for parathyroid adenoma, chemotherapy for malignancy).

2. Hypocalcemia

Hypocalcemia is defined as serum calcium levels <8.5 mg/dL, leading to neuromuscular excitability and other systemic effects.

Causes:

- **Hypoparathyroidism:**
    - Reduced PTH production due to surgery, autoimmune destruction, or genetic disorders.
    - **Key Lab Findings:**
        - Low calcium.
        - High phosphate.
        - Low PTH.
- **Vitamin D Deficiency:**
    - Caused by poor dietary intake, malabsorption, or inadequate sunlight exposure.
    - **Key Lab Findings:**
        - Low calcium.
        - Low phosphate.

- Low vitamin D.
- Elevated PTH (secondary hyperparathyroidism).
- **Chronic Kidney Disease (CKD):**
  - Impaired activation of vitamin D and phosphate retention, leading to secondary hyperparathyroidism.
  - **Key Lab Findings:**
    - Low calcium.
    - High phosphate.
    - Elevated PTH.

Clinical Features:

- Neuromuscular: Tetany, Chvostek's sign, Trousseau's sign, seizures.
- Cardiac: Prolonged QT interval.

Management:

- Acute: IV calcium gluconate for severe cases.
- Chronic: Oral calcium supplements and vitamin D analogs.
- Treat underlying cause (e.g., replace vitamin D, manage CKD).

Approach To Bone Disorders And Osteoporosis

Step 1: Evaluate the Bone Profile
- Check calcium, phosphate, ALP, vitamin D, and PTH levels.

- Determine if the pattern fits hyperparathyroidism, vitamin D deficiency, or renal osteodystrophy.

Step 2: Correlate with Clinical Features
- Assess for symptoms like bone pain, fractures, or deformities.
- Look for risk factors (e.g., age, corticosteroid use, immobility).

Step 3: Additional Investigations
- Bone mineral density (BMD) via dual-energy X-ray absorptiometry (DEXA) scan for osteoporosis.
- Imaging studies (e.g., X-rays for fractures or deformities).
- Biopsy in rare cases for conditions like Paget's disease.

Step 4: Management

Osteoporosis:

- **Definition:** Reduced bone density and increased fracture risk.
- **Risk Factors:** Age, postmenopausal status, corticosteroid use, smoking.
- **Diagnosis:**
    - T-score ≤ -2.5 on DEXA scan.
- **Treatment:**
    - Bisphosphonates (e.g., alendronate).
    - Denosumab for high-risk patients.

- Calcium and vitamin D supplementation.
- Lifestyle changes: Weight-bearing exercise, smoking cessation.

Other Bone Disorders:

- **Paget's Disease:**
    - Marked by disorganized bone remodeling.
    - Elevated ALP with normal calcium and phosphate.
    - Treat with bisphosphonates.
- **Osteomalacia:**
    - Softening of bones due to vitamin D deficiency.
    - Treat with vitamin D and calcium.

Case-Based Discussions

Case 1: Primary Hyperparathyroidism

- **Presentation:** Fatigue, frequent urination, bone pain.
- **Key Findings:**
    - Calcium: 11.2 mg/dL.
    - Phosphate: 2.2 mg/dL.
    - PTH: 85 pg/mL.
- **Diagnosis:** Primary hyperparathyroidism.
- **Management:** Parathyroidectomy for symptomatic patients or bisphosphonates for mild cases.

Case 2: Osteomalacia Due To Vitamin D Deficiency

- **Presentation:** Bone pain, muscle weakness, waddling gait.
- **Key Findings:**
    - Calcium: 8.0 mg/dL.
    - Phosphate: 2.0 mg/dL.
    - ALP: 200 U/L.
    - Vitamin D: 8 ng/mL.
- **Diagnosis:** Osteomalacia.
- **Management:** High-dose vitamin D and calcium supplementation.

CHAPTER 6: LIPID PROFILE

Components Of The Lipid Profile

1. Total Cholesterol (TC)
- **Normal Range:** Less than 200 mg/dL.
- **Clinical Significance:**
    - Represents the total amount of cholesterol in the blood, including both low-density lipoprotein (LDL), high-density lipoprotein (HDL), and very-low-density lipoprotein (VLDL) cholesterol.
    - Elevated levels of total cholesterol can indicate an increased risk of atherosclerosis and cardiovascular disease.
    - It is important to assess the individual components (LDL, HDL, and triglycerides) for a more accurate risk assessment.

2. Low-Density Lipoprotein (LDL) Cholesterol
- **Normal Range:** Less than 100 mg/dL (optimal); less than 70 mg/dL in high-risk patients.
- **Clinical Significance:**
    - Often referred to as "bad cholesterol," LDL is the primary carrier of cholesterol to peripheral tissues and is the major contributor to the development of atherosclerosis.
    - High levels of LDL are associated with

an increased risk of CVD, particularly in individuals with other risk factors like hypertension or diabetes.
- The goal of lipid-lowering therapy, especially with statins, is often to reduce LDL levels.

3. High-Density Lipoprotein (HDL) Cholesterol
- **Normal Range:** Greater than 40 mg/dL for men, greater than 50 mg/dL for women.
- **Clinical Significance:**
  - Known as "good cholesterol," HDL helps to remove excess cholesterol from peripheral tissues and transport it to the liver for excretion.
  - High levels of HDL are protective against cardiovascular disease as they promote reverse cholesterol transport.
  - Low HDL cholesterol levels are a significant risk factor for heart disease, and increasing HDL can help reduce risk.

4. Triglycerides
- **Normal Range:** Less than 150 mg/dL.
- **Clinical Significance:**
  - Triglycerides are the most common type of fat in the body and are a major energy source.
  - Elevated triglyceride levels are a significant risk factor for cardiovascular disease, especially when accompanied by high LDL or low HDL.
  - High triglycerides can be indicative of metabolic syndrome, obesity, uncontrolled

diabetes, or alcohol use.

Clinical Significance Of Abnormal Lipid Levels

1. Dyslipidemia

Dyslipidemia refers to abnormal levels of lipids in the blood, which may involve elevated levels of total cholesterol, LDL, triglycerides, and/or low levels of HDL.

Dyslipidemia can be categorized into two main types:

- **Primary (Familial) Dyslipidemia:**
    - Caused by genetic mutations that affect lipid metabolism.
    - Examples include familial hypercholesterolemia (elevated LDL) and familial combined hyperlipidemia (elevated triglycerides and cholesterol).
    - Individuals with primary dyslipidemia are at an increased risk for premature cardiovascular disease.
    - **Clinical Findings:**
        - High cholesterol levels from an early age.
        - Family history of early heart disease.
        - Tendon xanthomas (cholesterol deposits in tendons) in familial hypercholesterolemia.
- **Secondary Dyslipidemia:**
    - Caused by underlying conditions such as diabetes mellitus, hypothyroidism, kidney disease, or liver disease, as well as lifestyle factors like obesity, smoking, and excessive alcohol intake.

- **Conditions Associated with Secondary Dyslipidemia:**
  - **Diabetes Mellitus:** Elevated triglycerides and low HDL.
  - **Hypothyroidism:** Elevated total cholesterol and LDL.
  - **Chronic Kidney Disease:** Elevated triglycerides and LDL.
  - **Alcoholism:** Elevated triglycerides.

2. Risk Assessment for Cardiovascular Disease

The lipid profile is a crucial tool in assessing an individual's risk for cardiovascular diseases. The assessment should consider not only the lipid levels but also other risk factors, including age, sex, smoking, blood pressure, and presence of diabetes.

- **Total Cholesterol to HDL Ratio:**
  - This ratio is a useful predictor of cardiovascular risk. A ratio of greater than 5:1 indicates higher risk, while a ratio of 3.5:1 or lower is considered ideal.
  - **Clinical Application:**
    - If total cholesterol is elevated but HDL is also high, the risk may be less significant compared to high total cholesterol with low HDL.
    - Treatment targets should focus on reducing LDL levels and increasing HDL levels.
- **LDL Cholesterol Goal:**
  - The target LDL levels depend on the patient's risk profile. For high-risk patients (e.g., those with established cardiovascular disease or diabetes), the target LDL is often <70 mg/dL.

- For those at moderate risk, the target may be <100 mg/dL.
    - Statin therapy is commonly used to lower LDL cholesterol and reduce cardiovascular events.
- **Triglyceride Levels:**
    - Elevated triglycerides, especially above 500 mg/dL, increase the risk of pancreatitis and should be addressed promptly.
    - Triglycerides are also a marker of metabolic syndrome, which is associated with an increased risk of cardiovascular disease.

3. Management of Dyslipidemia Based on Lab Findings

The treatment of dyslipidemia involves both lifestyle modifications and pharmacologic interventions.

- **Lifestyle Modifications:**
    - **Dietary Changes:** Reducing saturated fats, trans fats, and cholesterol intake while increasing fiber, omega-3 fatty acids, and plant sterols.
    - **Exercise:** Regular aerobic exercise can increase HDL levels and decrease triglycerides.
    - **Weight Management:** Weight loss can reduce triglycerides and improve LDL/HDL ratios.
    - **Smoking Cessation:** Smoking lowers HDL cholesterol and increases the risk of atherosclerosis.
- **Pharmacologic Treatment:**
    - **Statins:** Statins are the first-line treatment for lowering LDL cholesterol. They work by inhibiting HMG-CoA reductase, which

reduces cholesterol synthesis in the liver.
- **Fibrates:** Fibrates, such as gemfibrozil and fenofibrate, are used to lower triglycerides and increase HDL levels.
- **Ezetimibe:** Ezetimibe inhibits cholesterol absorption in the intestines and is often added to statin therapy for further LDL reduction.
- **PCSK9 Inhibitors:** These newer agents are used for patients with familial hypercholesterolemia or those who do not achieve sufficient LDL lowering with statins.
- **Niacin:** Niacin (vitamin B3) can increase HDL levels, but its use is limited due to side effects like flushing and liver toxicity.

Differential Diagnosis Of Dyslipidemia

1. Primary Dyslipidemia:
- Familial Hypercholesterolemia: Elevated LDL, tendon xanthomas, early cardiovascular disease.
- Familial Combined Hyperlipidemia: Elevated total cholesterol and triglycerides, family history of premature cardiovascular disease.
- Familial Hypertriglyceridemia: Elevated triglycerides, increased risk of pancreatitis.

2. Secondary Dyslipidemia:
- **Diabetes Mellitus:** Elevated triglycerides, low HDL.
- **Hypothyroidism:** Elevated LDL, total cholesterol.
- **Chronic Kidney Disease:** Elevated LDL, triglycerides,

and low HDL.
- **Liver Disease:** Elevated triglycerides and LDL.

Case-Based Discussions

Case 1: Familial Hypercholesterolemia

- **Presentation:** A 45-year-old male with a family history of premature heart disease. He has tendon xanthomas and an elevated LDL of 230 mg/dL.
- **Diagnosis:** Familial hypercholesterolemia.
- **Management:** Statin therapy to lower LDL and reduce cardiovascular risk. Consideration of genetic testing for familial hypercholesterolemia.

Case 2: Metabolic Syndrome

- **Presentation:** A 50-year-old female with abdominal obesity, hypertension, elevated triglycerides (250 mg/dL), and low HDL (35 mg/dL).
- **Diagnosis:** Metabolic syndrome, with associated dyslipidemia.
- **Management:** Lifestyle changes (diet and exercise), metformin or other medications to improve insulin sensitivity, and statins to reduce cardiovascular risk.

CHAPTER 7: THYROID FUNCTION TESTS

Key Tests In Thyroid Function Evaluation

1. Thyroid Stimulating Hormone (Tsh)

- **Normal Range:** 0.4 to 4.0 mIU/L (varies slightly by laboratory).
- **Clinical Significance:**
    - TSH is produced by the pituitary gland and stimulates the thyroid gland to produce thyroid hormones (T4 and T3).
    - It is the most sensitive test for detecting thyroid dysfunction and is often the first test ordered.
    - High levels of TSH typically indicate hypothyroidism (underactive thyroid), while low levels suggest hyperthyroidism (overactive thyroid).
    - **Note:** TSH levels may be abnormal in non-thyroidal illness syndrome (euthyroid sick syndrome), where the TSH may be low despite a normal thyroid gland.

2. Free Thyroxine (Free T4)

- **Normal Range:** 0.8 to 1.8 ng/dL (varies by laboratory).

- **Clinical Significance:**
    - Free T4 is the unbound and biologically active form of thyroid hormone, representing the majority of circulating thyroid hormone.
    - Low levels of free T4 are characteristic of hypothyroidism, whereas elevated levels indicate hyperthyroidism.
    - Free T4 levels should always be interpreted in conjunction with TSH, as abnormalities in T4 levels can indicate primary thyroid dysfunction (disease of the thyroid gland itself) or secondary hypothyroidism (pituitary or hypothalamic dysfunction).

3. Free Triiodothyronine (Free T3)

- **Normal Range:** 2.3 to 4.2 pg/mL.
- **Clinical Significance:**
    - Free T3 is the active form of thyroid hormone and is responsible for most of the metabolic effects of thyroid hormones.
    - T3 levels are often elevated in hyperthyroidism and can provide additional diagnostic information in certain clinical scenarios.
    - In some cases of hyperthyroidism (such as in Graves' disease), T3 may be elevated disproportionately to T4, a condition known as "T3 toxicosis."
    - Free T3 levels are less commonly measured in routine thyroid testing, as free T4 and TSH are usually sufficient for diagnosing thyroid dysfunction.

4. Thyroid Antibodies

- **Types of Antibodies:**
    - **Anti-thyroid peroxidase (anti-TPO) antibodies**: These antibodies target thyroid peroxidase, an enzyme involved in thyroid hormone synthesis. Elevated levels are commonly seen in Hashimoto's thyroiditis.
    - **Anti-thyroglobulin antibodies**: These antibodies target thyroglobulin, a protein produced by the thyroid gland. Elevated levels may indicate autoimmune thyroid disease, particularly in Hashimoto's thyroiditis.
    - **Thyroid stimulating immunoglobulins (TSI)**: These antibodies stimulate the thyroid, leading to hyperthyroidism, and are typically present in Graves' disease.

Interpretation Of Thyroid Function Tests

1. Hypothyroidism Vs. Hyperthyroidism

- **Hypothyroidism:**
    - **Primary Hypothyroidism:** High TSH with low free T4. This occurs when the thyroid gland is not producing enough thyroid hormones, leading to compensatory elevation in TSH.
    - **Secondary Hypothyroidism:** Low TSH and low free T4. This occurs due to pituitary or hypothalamic dysfunction, where there is inadequate stimulation of the thyroid gland.

- **Clinical Features of Hypothyroidism:** Fatigue, weight gain, cold intolerance, constipation, depression, and dry skin.
- **Hyperthyroidism:**
  - **Primary Hyperthyroidism:** Low TSH with high free T4 and/or free T3. This indicates that the thyroid gland is overactive, producing excess thyroid hormones.
  - **Secondary Hyperthyroidism:** High TSH with high free T4 and free T3. This occurs when there is a pituitary adenoma secreting excess TSH, leading to overstimulation of the thyroid.
  - **Clinical Features of Hyperthyroidism:** Weight loss, tremors, palpitations, heat intolerance, increased sweating, and nervousness.

2. Subclinical Thyroid Dysfunction

- **Subclinical Hypothyroidism:**
  - Characterized by an elevated TSH (typically > 4.0 mIU/L) with normal free T4 and free T3.
  - It may occur in the early stages of autoimmune thyroid disease or in response to factors such as iodine deficiency or non-thyroidal illness syndrome.
  - Often asymptomatic, but may progress to overt hypothyroidism over time.
  - Treatment is generally not recommended unless there are symptoms or the TSH is very elevated (>10 mIU/L).
- **Subclinical Hyperthyroidism:**

- Characterized by a low TSH with normal free T4 and free T3 levels.
- It may occur due to early Graves' disease, thyroid autonomy (e.g., toxic multinodular goiter), or as a result of medications like thyroid hormone replacement therapy.
- While generally asymptomatic, there is an increased risk of atrial fibrillation, osteoporosis, and other cardiovascular complications.

Autoimmune Thyroid Diseases

1. Hashimoto's Thyroiditis (Chronic Lymphocytic Thyroiditis)

- **Cause:** Hashimoto's thyroiditis is the most common cause of hypothyroidism in iodine-sufficient areas. It is characterized by the destruction of the thyroid gland by autoimmune processes.
- **Laboratory Findings:**
    - Elevated anti-TPO and/or anti-thyroglobulin antibodies.
    - High TSH and low free T4 (hypothyroidism).
    - **Clinical Features:** Fatigue, cold intolerance, weight gain, and goiter.
    - **Management:** Levothyroxine replacement is the mainstay of treatment.

2. Graves' Disease

- **Cause:** Graves' disease is the most common cause

of hyperthyroidism, characterized by the production of thyroid-stimulating immunoglobulins (TSI), which stimulate the thyroid gland to produce excess thyroid hormones.

- **Laboratory Findings:**
    - Elevated TSI and low TSH.
    - High free T4 and free T3 (hyperthyroidism).
    - **Clinical Features:** Weight loss, heat intolerance, palpitations, and exophthalmos (bulging eyes).
    - **Management:** Antithyroid medications (e.g., methimazole), radioactive iodine therapy, or thyroidectomy.

Special Scenarios

1. Pregnancy And Thyroid Function

During pregnancy, thyroid hormone levels undergo physiological changes.

The increased production of estrogen leads to an increase in thyroid-binding globulin (TBG), which can affect the total thyroid hormone levels but does not typically affect the free T4 and free T3 levels. Proper thyroid function is crucial for fetal development, particularly for brain development.

- **First Trimester:** TSH levels may decrease slightly due to the increased hCG (human chorionic gonadotropin) levels, which can stimulate the thyroid gland.
- **Hypothyroidism in Pregnancy:** Must be promptly treated with levothyroxine to ensure adequate fetal development and avoid complications such as miscarriage or preterm delivery.
- **Hyperthyroidism in Pregnancy:** Can be caused by Graves' disease or pregnancy-induced hyperthyroidism. Treatment should be cautious, as some antithyroid medications can cross the placenta.

2. Non-Thyroidal Illness Syndrome (Ntis)

NTIS, also known as euthyroid sick syndrome, is a condition in which thyroid function tests are abnormal in the context of non-thyroidal illness (e.g., sepsis, trauma, or severe chronic illness).

In NTIS, TSH may be low or normal, and free T4 and T3 may be low.

This is a physiological response to illness and does not require treatment with thyroid hormones.

The changes in thyroid function are usually reversible once the underlying illness is treated.

Case-Based Discussions

Case 1: A 35-Year-Old Woman With Weight Gain, Fatigue, And Constipation

- **Lab Results:** High TSH, low free T4, elevated anti-TPO antibodies.
- **Diagnosis:** Hashimoto's thyroiditis (primary hypothyroidism).
- **Management:** Levothyroxine therapy.

Case 2: A 45-Year-Old Man With Weight Loss, Palpitations, And Anxiety

- **Lab Results:** Low TSH, high free T4, elevated TSI antibodies.
- **Diagnosis:** Graves' disease (hyperthyroidism).
- **Management:** Antithyroid medication or radioactive iodine therapy.

CHAPTER 8: INFLAMMATORY MARKERS

Key Inflammatory Markers

1. C-Reactive Protein (Crp)

- **Normal Range:** < 10 mg/L (varies by laboratory).
- **Clinical Significance:**
    - CRP is an acute-phase reactant, produced by the liver in response to cytokine release (primarily interleukin-6) during inflammation.
    - It rises quickly in response to infection, injury, or inflammation, and its levels correlate with the severity of inflammation.
    - CRP is widely used for assessing inflammation and monitoring the response to treatment, especially in infections and autoimmune diseases.
    - It is also used to monitor disease activity in conditions like rheumatoid arthritis, inflammatory bowel disease, and vasculitis.
    - **Advantages:** CRP levels rise rapidly (within 6-12 hours of inflammation) and return to baseline quickly once the underlying condition resolves, making it a useful marker for tracking disease progression and treatment efficacy.

2. Erythrocyte Sedimentation Rate (Esr)

- **Normal Range:**
  - Men: 0-15 mm/hour.
  - Women: 0-20 mm/hour.
- **Clinical Significance:**
  - ESR is a nonspecific test that measures the rate at which red blood cells settle in a tube of blood over an hour. The rate of sedimentation increases in the presence of acute-phase reactants, such as fibrinogen, that cause red blood cells to aggregate.
  - Although it is an older test, ESR remains useful in monitoring inflammatory diseases, particularly in conditions like systemic lupus erythematosus (SLE), temporal arteritis, and rheumatoid arthritis.
  - ESR tends to rise more slowly than CRP and remains elevated longer even after the resolution of inflammation. This makes it useful for assessing chronic inflammation or detecting relapsing diseases.
  - **Limitations:** ESR is influenced by various factors such as anemia, age, and pregnancy, which can lead to false positives or negatives.

3. Procalcitonin (Pct)

- **Normal Range:** < 0.1 ng/mL.
- **Clinical Significance:**
  - Procalcitonin is a precursor of the hormone calcitonin, which is produced in response to

bacterial infections. Unlike CRP, procalcitonin levels rise specifically in response to bacterial infections, making it a more specific marker for diagnosing bacterial sepsis or pneumonia.
- PCT levels can help differentiate bacterial infections from viral or inflammatory causes of fever.
- It is particularly useful in sepsis, guiding treatment decisions and antibiotic stewardship. Elevated procalcitonin levels in patients with suspected infections can suggest the need for antibiotics, while low levels can suggest the absence of bacterial infection, potentially preventing unnecessary antibiotic use.
- **Advantages:** PCT is more specific to bacterial infections compared to CRP and ESR, and it can be used to assess the severity of infection and monitor treatment effectiveness.

4. Ferritin

- **Normal Range:**
    - Men: 24-336 ng/mL.
    - Women: 11-307 ng/mL.
- **Clinical Significance:**
    - Ferritin is a protein that stores iron in the body. Although primarily associated with iron status, ferritin is also an acute-phase reactant, meaning its levels increase during inflammation, infection, and malignancy.
    - Ferritin is particularly useful in diagnosing and monitoring conditions like hemochromatosis, anemia of chronic disease,

and iron deficiency anemia.
- Inflammation causes ferritin levels to rise, and extremely high levels can suggest systemic inflammation or malignancy (e.g., lymphoma, leukemia).
- **Limitations:** Elevated ferritin can also be seen in liver disease, alcohol consumption, and conditions with excess iron storage, so its interpretation must consider other clinical factors.

Utility In Acute And Chronic Inflammation

Inflammatory markers are essential for assessing both acute and chronic inflammation, as their levels reflect the intensity and duration of the inflammatory process.

Acute Inflammation:

- **Causes:** Infection (bacterial, viral), trauma, surgery, and tissue injury (e.g., myocardial infarction, burns).
- **Marker Changes:**
    - **CRP:** Rises quickly (within 6-12 hours) after an acute injury or infection and returns to normal within a few days to weeks once the inflammatory stimulus resolves.
    - **ESR:** Increases gradually and remains elevated for a longer period after the acute phase ends.
    - **Procalcitonin:** Rises significantly in bacterial infections and can help differentiate bacterial from viral infections.

- **Ferritin:** May be elevated in response to acute-phase reactions but is not as specific as CRP or procalcitonin for bacterial infections.

Chronic Inflammation:

- **Causes:** Chronic infections (e.g., tuberculosis, HIV), autoimmune diseases (e.g., rheumatoid arthritis, lupus), malignancies, and metabolic disorders (e.g., obesity, diabetes).
- **Marker Changes:**
    - **CRP:** Remains elevated in chronic inflammatory conditions, such as rheumatoid arthritis, Crohn's disease, and vasculitis.
    - **ESR:** Often markedly elevated in chronic inflammatory diseases and is used for monitoring disease activity over time.
    - **Procalcitonin:** Generally remains low in chronic inflammation unless there is a superimposed bacterial infection.
    - **Ferritin:** Chronic inflammation can cause ferritin levels to rise, especially in diseases such as rheumatoid arthritis, cancer, and liver disease.

Differentiating Infectious, Autoimmune, And Malignant Causes

Infectious Causes:

- **CRP:** Elevated in both bacterial and viral infections, but

tends to be higher in bacterial infections.
- **PCT:** Specifically elevated in bacterial infections, making it a useful marker for differentiating bacterial infections from viral or inflammatory causes.
- **ESR:** Can be elevated in infections, especially chronic infections like tuberculosis.
- **Ferritin:** Elevated in infections with systemic involvement (e.g., sepsis) but is not specific to infection.

Autoimmune Diseases:

- **CRP:** Often elevated in autoimmune conditions such as rheumatoid arthritis, lupus, and vasculitis, reflecting ongoing inflammation.
- **ESR:** A key marker in autoimmune diseases, with particularly high levels seen in conditions like temporal arteritis, rheumatoid arthritis, and systemic lupus erythematosus (SLE).
- **Procalcitonin:** Usually normal or low in autoimmune diseases unless there is an associated bacterial infection.
- **Ferritin:** Elevated in autoimmune diseases, particularly in rheumatoid arthritis and lupus, due to the acute-phase response.

Malignant Causes:

- **CRP:** Elevated in malignancies, particularly those with associated inflammation, such as lymphoma, lung cancer, and gastrointestinal cancers.
- **ESR:** Often elevated in malignancies like lymphoma and multiple myeloma. It is commonly used as a

prognostic marker in some cancers.
- **Procalcitonin:** May be elevated in malignancy if there is a secondary bacterial infection or sepsis.
- **Ferritin:** Extremely high levels of ferritin can suggest malignancy, particularly hematologic malignancies like lymphoma, leukemia, and metastatic cancer.

CLINICAL LABORATORY MEDICINE PEARLS

Case-Based Discussions

Case 1: A 72-Year-Old Woman With Fever, Weight Loss, And Night Sweats

- **Lab Results:**
    - CRP: 45 mg/L (high).
    - ESR: 80 mm/hour (elevated).
    - PCT: 0.1 ng/mL (normal).
    - Ferritin: 600 ng/mL (elevated).
- **Diagnosis:** Likely malignancy (e.g., lymphoma or metastatic cancer). The elevated CRP, ESR, and ferritin suggest an inflammatory process, and the normal procalcitonin level rules out bacterial infection. Further imaging and biopsy are warranted.

Case 2: A 34-Year-Old Man With Joint Pain, Morning Stiffness, And Fatigue

- **Lab Results:**
    - CRP: 30 mg/L (elevated).
    - ESR: 70 mm/hour (elevated).
    - PCT: 0.05 ng/mL (low).
    - Ferritin: 350 ng/mL (elevated).
- **Diagnosis:** Likely autoimmune disease (e.g., rheumatoid arthritis). The elevated CRP and ESR are typical of systemic inflammation in autoimmune diseases. The low procalcitonin level suggests that a bacterial infection is unlikely. Further autoimmune markers, such as rheumatoid factor (RF) or anti-CCP antibodies, would help confirm the diagnosis.

CHAPTER 9: COAGULATION PROFILES

Key Coagulation Markers

1. Prothrombin Time (Pt)

- **Normal Range:** 11-13 seconds (varies by laboratory).
- **Clinical Significance:**
    - PT measures the time it takes for blood to clot after adding a reagent that activates the extrinsic pathway of coagulation (mainly involving factor VII).
    - It is used to assess the activity of several clotting factors (I, II, V, VII, and X), which are produced in the liver.
    - PT is commonly used to monitor patients on warfarin therapy (coumarin anticoagulants).
    - Prolonged PT can indicate liver dysfunction, vitamin K deficiency, or the presence of inhibitors such as anticoagulants.

2. International Normalized Ratio (Inr)

- **Normal Range:** 0.8-1.1 (varies by laboratory).
- **Clinical Significance:**
    - INR is a standardized version of PT that compensates for variations in laboratory

testing methods, allowing for consistency in monitoring anticoagulation therapy, particularly in patients on warfarin.
- The INR is typically aimed at a therapeutic range of 2.0-3.0 for patients on warfarin therapy.
- Prolonged INR can indicate over-anticoagulation or liver disease, and very low INR can suggest a hypercoagulable state.

3. Activated Partial Thromboplastin Time (Aptt)

- **Normal Range:** 25-35 seconds (varies by laboratory).
- **Clinical Significance:**
    - aPTT evaluates the intrinsic and common pathways of the coagulation cascade (factors XII, XI, IX, VIII, X, V, II, and I).
    - It is used to monitor patients on heparin therapy (unfractionated or low-molecular-weight heparins).
    - Prolonged aPTT may suggest the presence of clotting factor deficiencies, presence of lupus anticoagulant, or anticoagulant therapy (e.g., heparin).

4. D-Dimer

- **Normal Range:** < 0.5 µg/mL or < 250 ng/mL FEU (varies by laboratory).
- **Clinical Significance:**
    - D-dimer is a degradation product of cross-linked fibrin, which is produced when a clot is broken down by fibrinolysis.

- Elevated D-dimer levels indicate the presence of abnormal clotting and fibrinolysis, suggesting conditions such as deep vein thrombosis (DVT), pulmonary embolism (PE), disseminated intravascular coagulation (DIC), or significant trauma.
- D-dimer is particularly useful in the diagnosis of venous thromboembolism (VTE), although it is not specific and can be elevated in other conditions like pregnancy, malignancy, and inflammation.

5. Fibrinogen

- **Normal Range:** 200-400 mg/dL (varies by laboratory).
- **Clinical Significance:**
  - Fibrinogen is a plasma protein produced by the liver, and it is the precursor to fibrin, which forms the mesh of a blood clot.
  - Low fibrinogen levels can suggest consumptive coagulopathy, such as in DIC, or liver disease, whereas elevated fibrinogen levels may indicate an acute-phase reaction or inflammatory states, including infections or trauma.

Interpretation Of Coagulation Tests

Bleeding Disorders

1. **Hemophilia**
   - **Clinical Significance:**

- Hemophilia A and B are X-linked recessive bleeding disorders due to deficiencies in clotting factors VIII and IX, respectively.
- **Lab Findings:**
  - **PT/INR:** Normal (extrinsic pathway is unaffected).
  - **aPTT:** Prolonged (intrinsic pathway is affected).
  - **Fibrinogen/D-dimer:** Normal in hemophilia.
- **Diagnosis:** Genetic testing for factor VIII or IX deficiency is definitive.

2. **Von Willebrand Disease (vWD)**
   - Clinical Significance:
     - vWD is a hereditary bleeding disorder caused by a deficiency or dysfunction of von Willebrand factor, which is crucial for platelet adhesion and the stabilization of factor VIII.
     - **Lab Findings:**
       - **PT:** Normal.
       - **aPTT:** Prolonged (due to low factor VIII).
       - **D-dimer/Fibrinogen:** Normal.
     - **Diagnosis:** A multimodal approach, including bleeding history, von Willebrand factor antigen, and activity assays.

3. **Liver Disease**
   - Clinical Significance:

- The liver produces many of the coagulation factors. In liver failure, there is a deficiency of clotting factors, leading to coagulopathy.
- **Lab Findings:**
  - **PT/INR:** Prolonged (because of decreased production of clotting factors).
  - **aPTT:** Prolonged (affecting both the intrinsic and common pathways).
  - **Fibrinogen:** Decreased in severe liver disease.
- **Diagnosis:** Clinical findings (jaundice, hepatomegaly) and liver function tests (bilirubin, ALT/AST) are used alongside coagulation tests to confirm liver dysfunction.

Hypercoagulable States

1. **Disseminated Intravascular Coagulation (DIC)**
   - **Clinical Significance:**
     - DIC is a severe, life-threatening condition characterized by widespread activation of the clotting cascade, leading to the formation of microthrombi and consumption of clotting factors, resulting in bleeding.
   - **Lab Findings:**
     - **PT/INR:** Prolonged (due to consumption of clotting factors).
     - **aPTT:** Prolonged.

- **D-dimer:** Markedly elevated (reflecting ongoing fibrinolysis).
- **Fibrinogen:** Decreased (consumed in clot formation).
- **Diagnosis:** Clinical presentation (sepsis, trauma, malignancy) along with lab findings is crucial.

2. **Antiphospholipid Syndrome (APS)**
   - **Clinical Significance:**
     - APS is an autoimmune disorder characterized by the presence of antiphospholipid antibodies, leading to an increased risk of venous and arterial thrombosis, and pregnancy complications.
   - **Lab Findings:**
     - **PT/INR:** May be normal or prolonged.
     - **aPTT:** Prolonged (due to the lupus anticoagulant, an antiphospholipid antibody).
     - **D-dimer:** May be elevated in thrombosis.
     - **Fibrinogen:** May be elevated in acute thrombosis.
   - **Diagnosis:** Positive lupus anticoagulant, anticardiolipin antibodies, or anti-β2-glycoprotein I antibodies in the context of clinical symptoms.

Case-Based Applications

Case 1: A 45-Year-Old Man With Spontaneous Bleeding After Dental Surgery

- **Lab Results:**
    - PT: 12.5 seconds (normal).
    - INR: 1.0 (normal).
    - aPTT: 48 seconds (prolonged).
    - Fibrinogen: 350 mg/dL (normal).
- **Diagnosis:** The prolonged aPTT suggests an intrinsic pathway defect, possibly hemophilia. A history of easy bruising or prolonged bleeding after minor injuries would support this. Factor VIII or IX assay is needed for confirmation.

Case 2: A 28-Year-Old Woman With Recurrent Miscarriages

- **Lab Results:**
    - PT: 11 seconds (normal).
    - INR: 1.1 (normal).
    - aPTT: 40 seconds (prolonged).
    - D-dimer: Elevated.
    - Lupus anticoagulant: Positive.
- **Diagnosis:** Antiphospholipid syndrome (APS) is likely, given the positive lupus anticoagulant and clinical history of recurrent pregnancy loss. Further testing for antiphospholipid antibodies (anticardiolipin, anti-β2-

glycoprotein) is indicated for confirmation.

Case 3: A 65-Year-Old Woman With Jaundice And Easy Bruising

- **Lab Results:**
    - PT: 19 seconds (prolonged).
    - INR: 1.8 (elevated).
    - aPTT: 50 seconds (prolonged).
    - Fibrinogen: 120 mg/dL (low).
    - D-dimer: Elevated.
- **Diagnosis:** Liver disease with associated coagulopathy is the most likely diagnosis, given the elevated PT/INR and prolonged aPTT. Further liver function tests (ALT, AST, bilirubin) and imaging (ultrasound, CT) are necessary to evaluate for cirrhosis or liver failure.

CHAPTER 10: ADVANCED BIOCHEMICAL TESTS

1. Tumor Markers

Tumor markers are substances that are produced by tumors or by the body in response to cancer. They are used in oncology for screening, diagnosis, monitoring treatment response, and detecting recurrence. While they are not definitive on their own, elevated or decreased levels of certain tumor markers can provide important clues about the presence of malignancy.

1.1 Prostate-Specific Antigen (Psa)

- **Normal Range:** < 4 ng/mL (though reference ranges may vary based on age and other factors).
- **Clinical Significance:**
  - PSA is a glycoprotein produced by the prostate gland and is most commonly used for the detection of prostate cancer.
  - **Elevated PSA levels** may indicate prostate cancer, benign prostatic hyperplasia (BPH), or prostatitis.
  - PSA is useful in monitoring treatment response and detecting recurrence after prostate cancer treatment. However, PSA levels may be elevated in non-cancerous conditions such as BPH, urinary tract infections, and recent prostate manipulation (e.g., digital rectal exam or biopsy).

- **Limitations:** PSA is not a perfect screening tool, as it can give false positives (in non-cancer conditions) and false negatives (in early-stage cancers). Additionally, elevated PSA does not confirm cancer and requires further evaluation (e.g., biopsy).

1.2 Cancer Antigen 125 (Ca-125)

- **Normal Range:** < 35 U/mL (varies by laboratory).
- **Clinical Significance:**
    - CA-125 is a protein expressed by ovarian cancer cells and is primarily used to monitor ovarian cancer.
    - **Elevated levels** can be found in ovarian cancer, endometriosis, fibroids, pelvic inflammatory disease, and even in healthy menstruating women.
    - CA-125 is useful for monitoring the response to treatment and detecting recurrence in patients with known ovarian cancer.
    - **Limitations:** CA-125 is not specific for ovarian cancer and can be elevated in a variety of non-malignant conditions, limiting its utility as a screening tool in asymptomatic individuals.

1.3 Alpha-Fetoprotein (Afp)

- **Normal Range:** < 10 ng/mL in adults (varies by laboratory).
- **Clinical Significance:**
    - AFP is a glycoprotein produced by the

fetal liver and yolk sac. In adults, elevated AFP levels are associated with liver malignancies (e.g., hepatocellular carcinoma) and testicular cancer.
- **Elevated AFP** levels are seen in hepatocellular carcinoma, certain germ cell tumors, and other liver diseases like cirrhosis and hepatitis.
- AFP is also used for monitoring treatment response and detecting recurrence in hepatocellular carcinoma.
- **Limitations:** AFP can be elevated in non-cancerous liver diseases (e.g., cirrhosis, hepatitis), limiting its specificity for cancer detection.

2. Enzymes

Enzymes are proteins that catalyze biochemical reactions in the body. Elevated or decreased levels of certain enzymes can indicate organ dysfunction, injury, or disease. Some enzymes are specific to particular organs, while others may be elevated in a variety of conditions.

2.1 Amylase

- **Normal Range:** 23-85 U/L (varies by laboratory).
- **Clinical Significance:**
    - Amylase is an enzyme secreted by the pancreas and salivary glands that helps digest carbohydrates.
    - **Elevated amylase** is most commonly seen in pancreatitis, but it can also be elevated in conditions like salivary gland infections,

peptic ulcer disease, and bowel obstruction.
- **Limitations:** Amylase levels can be influenced by several factors, and a single elevated level is not diagnostic of pancreatitis. Other conditions, including gastrointestinal issues and renal failure, may also elevate amylase.

2.2 Lipase

- **Normal Range:** 10-140 U/L (varies by laboratory).
- **Clinical Significance:**
    - Lipase is an enzyme produced by the pancreas that breaks down fats.
    - **Elevated lipase** is a more specific indicator of pancreatitis compared to amylase. Lipase levels are usually significantly elevated in acute pancreatitis and can remain elevated longer than amylase.
    - **Limitations:** Although lipase is more specific than amylase, it can still be elevated in other conditions like gastrointestinal perforations, renal failure, and certain medications.

3. Specialized Tests

These tests measure specific compounds or physiological markers that provide valuable information about organ function, metabolic states, or disease conditions.

3.1 Lactate

- **Normal Range:** 0.5-2.2 mmol/L (varies by laboratory).
- **Clinical Significance:**
    - Lactate is produced during anaerobic metabolism, and elevated lactate levels indicate tissue hypoxia, sepsis, or metabolic disturbances.
    - **Elevated lactate** can suggest conditions like sepsis, shock, severe hypoxia, ischemia, and mitochondrial disorders. It is often used in critically ill patients to assess metabolic status and guide treatment.
    - **Limitations:** Lactate levels can be influenced by several factors, including exercise, drugs, and liver or renal failure. Elevated lactate alone is not diagnostic and requires clinical correlation.

3.2 Ammonia

- **Normal Range:** 15-45 µg/dL (varies by laboratory).
- **Clinical Significance:**
    - Ammonia is a waste product produced during protein metabolism and is primarily processed by the liver. Elevated ammonia levels are indicative of liver dysfunction or

failure.
- **Elevated ammonia** is seen in conditions like hepatic encephalopathy, cirrhosis, and urea cycle disorders.
- **Limitations:** Ammonia levels may fluctuate, and elevations are not always specific to liver disease. Blood sample handling is important, as ammonia levels can rise quickly after collection.

3.3 Serum Osmolality

- **Normal Range:** 275-295 mOsm/kg (varies by laboratory).
- **Clinical Significance:**
    - Serum osmolality measures the concentration of solutes in the blood, including sodium, glucose, urea, and other electrolytes.
    - **Elevated osmolality** can be seen in hypernatremia, dehydration, or excessive intake of osmotically active substances (e.g., mannitol or alcohol).
    - **Low osmolality** can be indicative of conditions like hyponatremia, overhydration, or the syndrome of inappropriate antidiuretic hormone (SIADH).
    - **Limitations:** Serum osmolality can be influenced by factors such as blood glucose and urea levels, and it is usually used in conjunction with other tests to determine the underlying cause of the abnormality.

Clinical Contexts And Limitations

Advanced biochemical tests can provide valuable diagnostic information, but they should be interpreted in the context of the patient's clinical presentation.

The limitations of these tests include:

1. **False positives and false negatives:** Many tests, such as tumor markers, can be elevated in non-malignant conditions, and the presence of a tumor marker does not always correlate with the presence of cancer. Similarly, normal levels do not rule out disease.
2. **Influence of comorbid conditions:** Conditions such as liver disease, renal failure, and inflammation can alter the levels of enzymes and other biochemical markers.
3. **Need for confirmatory tests:** Advanced biochemical tests often require further diagnostic work-up, including imaging, biopsy, or genetic testing, for a definitive diagnosis.
4. **Interference by medications:** Some medications, such as statins, anticoagulants, and corticosteroids, can affect enzyme and tumor marker levels.

CHAPTER 11: INTEGRATING LABORATORY RESULTS WITH CLINICAL CONTEXT

1. Using Lab Results In Diagnostic Algorithms

1.1 Diagnostic Algorithms In Medicine

- **Stepwise Approach**: A common method in integrating lab results is using a stepwise approach, where each clinical and laboratory finding helps narrow down the differential diagnosis. For example, if a patient presents with fatigue and pallor, a Full Blood Count (FBC) is performed to assess for anemia. If the hemoglobin is low, further testing (such as a reticulocyte count, iron studies, or vitamin B12 levels) helps differentiate between different causes of anemia (e.g., iron deficiency, vitamin B12 deficiency, or chronic disease).
- **Pattern Recognition**: Many conditions have characteristic patterns of lab findings that can be identified through algorithms. For instance, in suspected liver disease, the pattern of enzyme elevation (AST, ALT, ALP, GGT) and bilirubin levels can indicate whether the injury is hepatocellular (e.g., viral hepatitis) or cholestatic (e.g., gallstones).
- **Confirmatory Testing**: Once a likely diagnosis is established, lab results often prompt further confirmatory tests. For instance, a positive HIV test

result leads to confirmatory viral load and CD4 count measurements, while a suspected myocardial infarction based on elevated troponins would prompt further cardiac imaging (e.g., echocardiogram, angiography) to assess the extent of damage.

1.2 The Role Of Lab Results In Differential Diagnosis

- **Narrowing the Differential**: Laboratory results help narrow down the list of possible diagnoses by either confirming or eliminating certain conditions. For instance, an elevated white blood cell count with a left shift suggests an infection, while a negative result for bacterial cultures may point to viral causes, such as influenza or Epstein-Barr virus.
- **Thresholds and Decision Points**: Diagnostic algorithms use thresholds to determine the likelihood of various diagnoses. For example, an elevated troponin level above a certain threshold is highly indicative of acute myocardial infarction, guiding the clinician toward cardiology consultation and intervention.
- **Guiding Treatment**: Laboratory tests, when interpreted correctly, can help guide treatment decisions. For example, elevated glucose levels in a diabetic patient may prompt adjustments in insulin therapy, or an elevated INR in a patient on warfarin may guide a temporary change in anticoagulation strategy.

2. Combining Lab Findings With Imaging And Clinical Signs

2.1 Imaging And Clinical Signs In Context

- **Imaging Studies**: Imaging modalities such as X-rays, CT scans, MRI, and ultrasound complement laboratory results in providing a more complete picture of the patient's condition. For example, in a patient with elevated liver enzymes, imaging studies like ultrasound or CT may help identify liver lesions, cirrhosis, or bile duct obstruction, allowing for more precise diagnosis (e.g., hepatocellular carcinoma vs. benign fatty liver).
- **Clinical Signs and Symptoms**: Clinical examination findings provide essential clues that guide lab interpretation. For instance, a patient presenting with jaundice and elevated bilirubin may have liver disease, but the presence of ascites and spider nevi may point to cirrhosis rather than acute hepatitis.
- **Case Example**: In a patient with chest pain, elevated troponins, and ST elevation on an EKG, the lab findings combined with clinical signs and imaging (such as coronary angiography) will confirm the diagnosis of acute myocardial infarction and guide management toward reperfusion therapy.

2.2 Correlation Between Lab Results And Clinical Context

- **Matching Lab Findings with Symptoms**: It's essential to correlate lab results with the patient's history and symptoms. For example, in a patient with fatigue, pallor, and a low hemoglobin level, anemia is likely. However, additional tests like iron studies or vitamin B12 levels can help determine the cause of the anemia.

- **Epidemiological Factors**: Consider the patient's demographic and epidemiological context. A positive malaria test in a patient returning from sub-Saharan Africa is more likely to be accurate than in a patient who has never traveled outside their country.
- **Example in Endocrinology**: A patient with weight loss, tachycardia, and tremors with elevated free T4 and suppressed TSH likely has hyperthyroidism (possibly from Graves' disease), but this diagnosis must be confirmed with thyroid antibody testing and imaging studies (e.g., thyroid ultrasound or radioactive iodine uptake scan).

3. Avoiding Pitfalls In Interpretation

3.1 Pseudohyperkalemia

- **What It Is**: Pseudohyperkalemia occurs when blood samples are improperly handled, leading to falsely elevated potassium levels. This can occur if there is hemolysis of red blood cells during sample collection or transport, releasing intracellular potassium into the bloodstream.
- **Clinical Implication**: It's important to confirm elevated potassium levels with a repeat blood test, particularly in a patient without clinical signs of hyperkalemia (such as ECG changes, muscle weakness, or arrhythmias).
- **Prevention**: Proper collection and handling of samples, avoiding excessive fist-clenching during venipuncture, and immediate processing of blood samples can help prevent pseudohyperkalemia.

3.2 Lab Errors

- **Types of Errors**: Lab errors can occur due to faulty reagents, calibration issues, or mislabeling of samples. These errors can lead to inaccurate results that may mislead clinicians.
- **Clinical Implication**: Clinicians should always consider the possibility of lab errors, especially when the lab results do not align with clinical findings. If the clinical picture contradicts laboratory results, repeat testing or confirmation with a different test may be necessary.
- **Prevention**: Regular quality control measures, including verifying lab equipment calibration and participating in external proficiency testing, help minimize the risk of errors.

3.3 Physiological Variations

- **Factors Affecting Lab Results**: Many lab results can vary based on factors like age, sex, race, body mass index, and hydration status. For instance, serum creatinine may be lower in older adults due to decreased muscle mass, or a pregnant patient may have altered blood counts or liver function tests.
- **Clinical Implication**: These physiological variations should be considered when interpreting lab results. Age-related reference ranges should be applied to ensure that results are appropriately assessed in context.
- **Prevention**: Clinicians must be aware of these variations and use reference ranges that are appropriate for the patient's demographic.

3.4 False Positives And False Negatives

- **False Positives**: These occur when a test indicates the presence of a condition that is not actually present. For instance, an elevated D-dimer in a patient with no signs of clotting could be due to conditions like pregnancy, inflammation, or recent surgery.
- **False Negatives**: These occur when a test fails to detect a condition that is present. For example, a negative rapid strep test does not rule out streptococcal pharyngitis, especially in cases of low bacterial load.
- **Clinical Implication**: Both false positives and false negatives can lead to inappropriate treatment or missed diagnoses. It's essential to use confirmatory tests and integrate clinical signs and other diagnostic modalities.

ABOUT THE AUTHOR

Dr Essam Abdelhakim

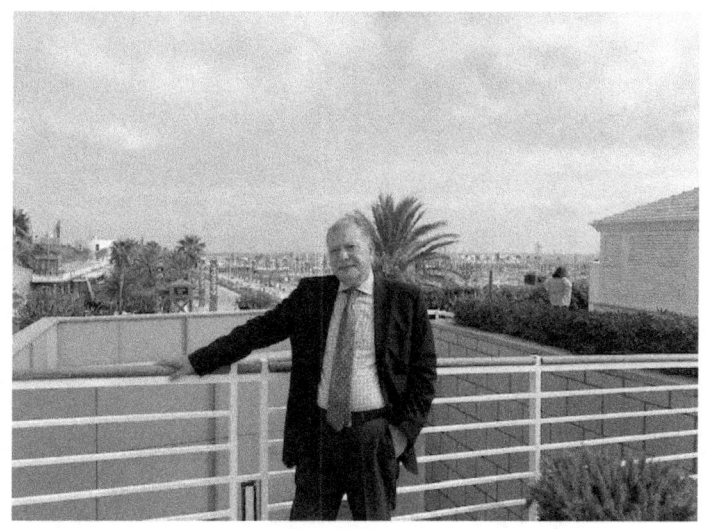

Senior Consultant and Expert in Medical Education

www.ingramcontent.com/pod-product-compliance
Lightning Source LLC
Chambersburg PA
CBHW071105240526
45469CB00006BD/2337